# Kaeleb's Dad

MICHAEL WALSH

Copyright © 2014 Michael Walsh
All rights reserved.

ISBN-10: 1500615927
ISBN-13: 978-1500615925

DEDICATION

This book is dedicated to my wife Debra and our two sons Chad and Justin who all contributed in teaching me what family and love are all about.

## CONTENTS

| | Acknowledgments | i |
|---|---|---|
| 1 | January 1982. Phoenix, Arizona | 1 |
| 2 | The First Month | 6 |
| 3 | Second Month | 14 |
| 4 | Third Month | 18 |
| 5 | Fourth Month | 22 |
| 6 | Fifth Month | 27 |
| 7 | Sixth Month | 32 |
| 8 | Seventh Month | 36 |
| 9 | Eighth Month | 40 |
| 10 | Ninth Month | 43 |
| 11 | Thirty-Two Years Later | 46 |
| | About the Author | 50 |
| | More Books | 51 |

# ACKNOWLEDGMENTS

When you experience something like the incidents in this book, you quickly realize that you could not do it alone.

I need to thank so many people for their help. I will try to do the list justice. First, I need to acknowledge the strength and courage of my wife, Debra Walsh; she was amazing during it all. Dr. Barry Fisher and his staff were outstanding through the whole thing. Our pediatrician was also there to support us every day.

There is no way to ever acknowledge the help and support other parents have given us. I clearly still remember Charlie and Julie Brown along with Mike and Summer Stacy being the main branches of support.

Two very kind people need to be thanked for helping me finish the second edition of *Kaeleb's Dad*, namely Christina Lane and my good friend and relative through marriage, Angela Harris. Thank you both for everything that you did to help me complete this story.

# 1 JANUARY 1982. PHOENIX, ARIZONA

There I was sitting in the courtyard of the Phoenix Baptist Hospital. I don't remember if the sun was shining, if it was cloudy, the colors around me or the chaos of hospital courtyard. But, what I do remember is staring blankly at the most beautiful woman I'd ever met. She just stood there by the door staring back at me.

She was dressed in a blue dress with a yellow belt, which proved to only further emphasize her thin shape. She weighed 110 pounds if she was lucky. Her dark-brown hair flowed to shoulder length with the right front combed back and then falling into silken waves. Her hazel eyes were penetrating when she looked at you on any given day but even more so now.

It was hard to believe that this woman had just given me an ultimatum. At least that was the way I interpreted it. For the words, "this baby is going to make it with or without you," had just come out of her mouth. We'd just found out that our son was diagnosed as a potential SIDS child and the terror of that message was tearing us apart. She knew the fears and pain that accompanied the loss of a child from SIDS. And now, we'd just learned that we *may* have to endure that pain and fear once more—but *she* had decided immediately that this wouldn't happen to our family again. My God, where did she get such courage and resolve?

At this point, I didn't know what to do. I walked up to her and hugged her, my mind was overwhelmed with anger at the world for our son's illness, fear at having to endure this once again, and *love*. We entered the hospital to meet with the doctor and discuss our son's illness. I don't remember noticing anything around me at all as we made our way through the hospital hallways to the doctor's office. I'm sure we performed the routine pleasantries before we sat to discuss our son's illness but...if so I don't remember. The first thing I do remember about this meeting is the doctor telling us that our son would quit breathing for longer than thirty seconds 30% of the time when he was sleeping.

Then the doctor escorted us to our son. There he was in the neo-natal intensive care unit waiting for us. You just knew that the doctor hated giving this kind of message to parents. I remember realizing that in some still active part of my brain. The doctor was shifting his weight from one foot to the other as he spoke. To me, it was all babble; the only parts I remembered, of the conversation, were that our child couldn't leave the hospital until we'd completed a course in infant CPR and been certified in it. They did have the ability to conduct the class and could certify us both right there in the hospital, we were informed as we followed him through the maze of hallways that lead to the neo-natal intensive care unit.

The doctor did ask, and I am not sure why, if we were willing to take the class. Without hesitation, my wife answered with "Yes." I don't remember if I made any response at all as I continued to gather my scattered emotions. But I do remember that before we went to the class, I finally managed to gather my wits and speak my first words of the afternoon. I asked the doctor if we could see our child before we took the class. His response was, "Of course, it would take them about an hour to get everything setup for us." He then led us to the glass crib the baby was lying in. As soon as we entered the room, something unusual happened. This one-month-old baby turned and looked at both of us.

Those big, brown eyes of his, they seemed to penetrate right through me. I could feel their warmth, anxiety, and love all the way through my body. This was the first time I'd experienced such unconditional love from a look. We both just stared at each other. I couldn't speak and he didn't know how. But he did speak to me, with warmth that I had never felt before.

The next thing that I remember was the nurse was coming to get us for the class. When the hour was over; it felt like we had just gotten there. This is where reality started to hit. We were informed, again, that the baby could not go home until we had been certified in infant CPR. Okay, alright. I felt some semblance of reality returning to my brain; it was time to get serious.

We were led off to CPR class. There we were introduced to the nurse leading the class. The nurse then proceeded to demonstrate the monitoring equipment that we'd be bringing home with our son. I'll admit that none of the equipment's aspects hit home with me, until we had to install it later. The nurse then demonstrated the alarm. THE LOUDEST AND MOST AWFUL IRRITATING TONE you'd ever heard came out of that little box. Of course we understood why it was so loud. That noise was set to wake up a city for good reason. The nurse explained to us that when the baby stopped breathing for longer than thirty seconds the alarm would go off. Once we understood that, it really didn't matter how loud it was. After her explanation of its purpose, we wanted to know everything we could about it.

The nurse then proceeded to tell us that we could never be further than TEN seconds away from the baby when he was sleeping. The reason for the TEN seconds was that we were supposed to let him bring himself out of an episode without our intervention. I remember my thought at that time was, if that noise didn't bring him back nothing would. The nurse then informed us that our next step was to call his name and tap his feet. All of this was to get him to bring himself back to normal breathing.

The last resort would be infant CPR. You really don't understand how fragile a baby's body is until you try to learn how to give it infant CPR. Learning how to place two fingers in the right place and supply the right amount of pressure was terrifying and just about doing me in. Over and over, I kept saying to myself, "I hope I never have to do this." Finally we passed certification. The anxiety that I was having during this course was obvious even to the nurse; she just kept saying to me, "You'll get it." And finally, I did. I think I got the whole process right once. And that was enough for her to let us take the baby home. I remember thinking again as she certified us, I hope that I never have to do this for real.

## 2 THE FIRST MONTH

On the way home from the hospital all kinds of thoughts were running through my head. Any and all scenery or traffic on that drive home totally escaped me; but somehow I managed to safely maneuver through the traffic at that time of day. But uppermost in my mind was that I just couldn't completely accept what we'd just gone through. This tiny, beautiful child couldn't have anything wrong with him, I kept thinking. I was in DENIAL. And deep down somewhere I knew that was going to have to change.

At home was my wife's oldest son, who was nine and a half years old at the time. For his age he was very mature. He had to be. He had lost a brother to SIDS at six months old, and he had learned to live with it. Or so he claimed. Before his youngest brother was born, he and I had been getting very close. We'd spend all of our time together. I felt like we'd finally gotten to a point where we were beginning to know each other well. And we truly enjoyed each other's company. Now, we had to tell him he might lose another brother. My heart broke at that thought and I knew that that conversation was not going to be easy.

When we got to the house, my wife asked me to stay in the car while she talked to our oldest son. I remember my immediate response was, "What if the baby quits breathing?"

She just looked at me calmly and said, "Put your hand lightly on his chest to make sure that he's breathing. And if he stops you know what to do. You've been trained." Yeah, I was trained. But I was nowhere near ready to do anything. But with a mixture of fear and almost overwhelming apprehension, I put my hand lightly on his chest and waited. It seemed as if she was gone forever.

And then, thankfully, she came out of the house with our oldest son following behind her. She then proceeded to tell me that our oldest son wanted to learn infant CPR too. That blew me away. But, the doctors did say that any member of our family was eligible to learn at any time. I'm not sure that they or I were ready for this innocent child to take on such responsibility; but I couldn't have been more proud of him than I was at that moment. And some far away part of my brain knew that letting him learn CPR may help him to deal with his brother's illness too; empower him in a way, help him to not feel so helpless.

Once we got the baby down for a nap, my wife decided that she needed a shower. I remember my response was, "Are you nuts! What if the baby quits breathing while you're in there?"

She calmly looked at me and said, "If you think I am not going to take a shower until he's outgrown the chance of having an episode, you have another thing coming. Besides, you've been trained; you know what to do if anything happens." I had to think about it. Some part of my rational brain must have been present because it shoved the fear aside and took over. She was right. So she went off to take her shower. Once she was in there, I immediately went to the baby's crib side and watched for his breathing with a single minded focus all the while she was in there. I remember thinking that that shower was the longest moments of my life. To this day, I don't think she knows about that and how scared, hopelessly scared, I was all the while she showered.

That night, I found myself repeating a prayer over and over to myself until I fell asleep. It went like this: *Please, dear Lord, please let little Justin (our youngest), Chad (our oldest), and Deb (my wife), be healthy and safe. Dear Lord, please! If you do I will thank you so much.*

This prayer I remember constantly repeating until I fell asleep every night for many, many nights. Praying felt a little strange for me at first and then it became a natural thing. You can never understand such overwhelming helplessness unless you've experienced it. I was afraid. Not just of losing baby Justin, but… of losing any of my family and I knew it.

It took a couple of days before we had our first incident. Time had allowed me to relax a little; obviously, I was getting overconfident. There's no way to explain the reaction you have at hearing that loud tone at 3:00 a.m. in the morning except **panic.** You can forget about waiting ten seconds to revive him. We were all by the side of the crib in less than two seconds. And forget that calling his name routine.

At that time of the morning, you only want that tone to stop. So you tap the baby's feet lightly until the tone goes off; signaling that he is breathing normally again. Somehow, you manage to take your panicked, shaky body back to bed and if you're lucky…you go back to sleep, if you can. It would sometimes take us hours to fall asleep. And getting up for work for 6:00 a.m. was often a chore beyond belief.

Fortunately, the people at my job were very understanding. So much so that they provided me with a beeper if anything happened and my wife called. That was something that I did not want to hear about. And you'd better believe that every time my wife did call, they all scrambled to get in contact with me. There was a bright spot though: she felt guilty about calling and asking me to pickup items at the store on the way home. My excitement about this didn't last long though; as she'd just wait until I got home and send me out to the store then.

It got to the point where we averaging three alarms a week. Unfortunately, it was always at 3:00 a.m. in the morning. I was spending fifty to sixty hours a week at work to hide from the activities at home. I didn't want to be there if anything happened to him. Somewhere deep inside I knew it was selfish; but I now know I was terrified. Terrified of the worst happening and…I didn't want to be there when it did.

My wife quickly amended her schedule when she realized what I was doing. Now, looking back, I know that she didn't want my fear…of what may happen, to stop me bonding with and loving my wonderful son. The next thing I knew I ended up babysitting while she'd go out shopping. What a rude awakening to reality. I had to learn how to deal with diapers *and* the monitor.

During this time, we were making weekly visits to the hospital for the baby's checkups and Theophelon shots. The theory behind the Theophelon was that it was like caffeine and it would allow the baby to get into a REM sleep, thus reducing the incidents. It was during one of these visits that our doctor asked if we'd be willing to work with other parents who had children with this illness. After thinking about it, we decided that it would help us as well as them in coping with the situation. Our doctor immediately introduced us to two other couples.

During that meeting, I remember our doctor asked all of us to form a support group for other families in our area that had children suspected of being SIDS candidates. Who could know how much that one suggestion would mean to us, and to the other parents of children with SIDS. There was no way of knowing how much benefit we would derive from that one suggestion. We agreed and then found out that there were 170 families involved with the SIDS support group throughout Arizona. That was unimaginable! One hundred and seventy families in Arizona alone were dealing with the same fear and terror that we were because of this illness.

Once we agreed, the doctor gave us another eye-opening number. He told us that the divorce rate among SIDS families was around 90%. His hope was that giving support to both parents would be beneficial in the effort to reduce this rate. I remembered thinking that he had to be kidding. If the other parents were anything like me and my wife, they weren't interested in being marriage counselors. They were only interested in whether their children could survive this illness and that's all.

As part of our organization, we had to give talks to visiting nurses and residents who wanted to learn as much as they could on the subject. It was during one of these talks that my wife just blew me away. In front of one hundred visiting nurses she stood up and started talking about being a mother of a SIDS child.

As I watched her, I kept asking myself, **what happened to the self-conscious woman I'd met who was so shy that she'd barely say one word to anyone?** This couldn't be that same woman. Here instead was a confident, opinionated speaker who was captivating her audience. Through my astonishment, I was again reminded of why I love her the way I do.

Let's see, we have the baby triggering his alarms three times a week and we're giving talks to the medical profession, what else could happen? Well, I found out. The local telephone company called my wife one day and asked if she would be willing to volunteer for a hotline service for people who had found out that their children were potential SIDS children. Needless to say, she agreed to it. So now, we also were getting phone calls all hours of the day and night. She was amazing; she would listen to them for hours. She'd never let them give up hope for their children.

It was also at this time that our doctor decided to tell us that he was writing a book on the subject of near-miss SIDS children, and he wanted to include our son's case in his book. We agreed; after all, it would give our son a chance to help other families in the future.

It was about this time that we remembered that

we wanted our child to be baptized. Now, both of us being Catholic, that wasn't a problem. But both of us having a previous marriage was, in the eyes of the church, a problem. The priest we went to see told us that we'd have to apply for annulment for our previous marriages. My response to him was that this child had nothing to do with our previous marriages and he had a right to be baptized. The priest finally gave in once he understood the family history. The day of the baptism was an interesting day. The priest was pouring water over our son's head during the ceremony when he, the baby, decided to take the towel out of the priest's hands and proceeded to let loose with some of loudest crying you've ever heard. It took the priest, the surrogate godfather, and the surrogate godmother in order to remove the towel from our son's hands. He proceeded to cry even louder after they did. It was at this point that my wife leaned over to me and said, "That's your son."

## 3 SECOND MONTH

The daily routine around our house was beginning to become clear about this time. We'd respond to the monitor at 3:00 a.m. in the morning and answer the hotline whenever there was a phone call.

It was also at this time that we started meeting with the other parent leaders of our support group to learn what our rolls would be. It didn't take long for us to realize that we were lucky on a couple of counts. First, our insurance company covered the monthly cost of the monitor as well as all the doctor's visits for our youngest son.

Needless to say, this was not the case for all the other parents. The more we researched it, the more we found out that we were exceptions to the rule. My wife quickly volunteered to contact the insurance companies to discuss the situation with them. Now this was interesting, they gave her every run-around you could think of, from passing her around to every member of their company to "accidently" hanging up on her.

That was a big mistake. Eventually, she would get to a VP or account executive and they would make the classic mistake. They would get so frustrated with her arguments that they would finally say, "After all, it is not a life-threatening situation." Once that was said it was like the heavens opened up and spewed forth their wrath. My wife was unstoppable and they had no other choice than to cave in and support the rental of the monitor for the families. It was a beautiful thing to watch.

The other thing that we found out was that 90% of potential SIDS children (at the time) had other complications. It normally ran between cystic fibrosis to epilepsy. So far we'd not seen any symptoms of either one with our youngest son though. It became clear to us that each child was unique in how they exhibited their symptoms.

One of the parents was more than willing to share the story of his youngest daughter. She'd regularly quit breathing during her naps. It was to the point that they had given her CPR once a week to revive her. It was during one of these episodes that the ambulance had to be called. Both of the parents thought they'd lost their child at this point. But the ambulance came and the baby was rushed to the hospital and revived.

About two hours later though, there was a knock at their door. The father answered it. There stood a police officer looking very sad and shifting his feet as he said, "We're very sorry about your little girl. But since a death was involved we need to fill out a police report."

The father immediately asked the officer, "Do you mean that little girl playing over there?"

The officer's jaw dropped and he couldn't believe it. It turned out that this child would get revived by the sound of the siren on the ambulance at a rate of once every two weeks.

The father then proceeded to tell us about the many times the police came to the house trying to charge him and his wife with child abuse. Obviously, this didn't hold up and they just didn't understand what was going on with the children. Education for the public quickly became a priority for him and he was very successful in that area.

During this time, the visiting nurses of Arizona contacted us and volunteered to babysit for any of our groups parents to allow them to have a night out once a week. This was a godsend for many of us. She also helped us to set up some research on SIDS and its known causes. At the time, there were two known causes: the first was that the brain was not developed enough to remind the infant to breath while they were asleep, the second was the lack of development of a certain muscle in the throat of the infant that would intermittently cause the infant to block the flow of oxygen to their lungs. The second of these two is what the doctors determined our son had. The trick now was to learn as much as we could about the subject. So we did.

It turns out that there is nothing you can do until the muscle is developed. Not what I wanted to hear.

Another interesting thing also happened during this time frame. A woman who was a friend of a co-worker volunteered to become infant CPR certified to babysit for our youngest son. Guess what? The doctors even let our oldest son become certified. I was amazed.

By the end of the month, our youngest son was getting pretty comfortable with his monitor and its associated cabling. So much so, in fact, that he would, when he wanted attention, pull on the cable until the alarm went off. We obviously came running too when he'd do this. He'd then proceed to smile and hand us the cable. To him, this was so fun; but for us, of course, it was no fun at all.

## 4 THIRD MONTH

It was about this time that our youngest son found his hands and feet; watching that experience was beautiful.

Once he found his appendages, he proceeded investigate how to use them. Now, that was an interesting time. He could now sit up and spend time in a different way with the family. Whenever he smiled, his whole body smiled with him. He smiled a lot.

During this time, his older brother and I played with him constantly and he loved it. This was also the time that I decided to grow a beard; purely out of laziness. The first time our youngest son noticed it, he just stared at it with a puzzled expression on his face. The next time he saw it he rubbed it with his hand. I remember laughing, as I thought he was trying to rub it off. Then the next thing I knew he had a hold of it on both sides and was proceeding to do chin ups with my beard. You want to talk about pain. Needless to say, once I got his hands out of my beard, that beard lasted all of five minutes; after that, the beard disappeared, never to return again.

After that experience, things seemed to calm down for a couple of days. Then one day, I came home and my wife was very distraught. When she finally told me why I couldn't believe it; according to her she'd put the baby down for his nap and forgotten to set the monitor. This meant that if he quit breathing during that time she'd never have known about it. She was beside herself. I told her not to worry about it; he was fine and just to **make** sure that she didn't do it again. I had to say that, she's my wife; but deep down I was just as terrified as her. The next day I came home and she said she did it again.

Now I was really getting concerned. I tried to think of all the possibilities why this could be happening: did she just forget, did the machine fail, or was she just thinking that she had set the monitor? When quizzed on this, she said she was positive that she had set it correctly. My response to her was to keep a close eye on it the next time when she put him down for a nap.

When I came home the next day, I couldn't believe what she was telling me. She'd put the baby down for his nap, turned the machine on, stepped out of the room, and sat on the stairs, where she could watch the monitor to make sure that it was still working. Then from within the crib a little hand had reached out and shut the monitor off. Mystery solved! You wouldn't believe how quickly that monitor was placed across the room.

It was also during this same time frame that one of the visiting nurses was coming to our home to monitor our youngest son's progress. He was doing great. At least as far I was concerned. My wife, however, was concerned. It seems that when she spoke to our youngest son he'd ignore her. She'd get no response at all from him.

This bothered her. She thought that he might be deaf, or at least losing his hearing. After all, the other potential SIDS children all had multiple things wrong with them. So this notion wasn't without merit. After talking to the visiting nurse they decided to have his hearing tested. The doctors were a little concerned that a child his age would be exhibiting hearing loss but they agreed. They'd learned a long time ago that it wasn't good to argue with my wife when she was upset. So the hearing tests were conducted and the doctor said he'd send the results along with the visiting nurse within two weeks.

Well, those two weeks seemed to take forever. My wife was going crazy waiting for the results. Then the visiting nurse finally came. It turned out that the baby was fine. He'd simply decided to ignore any sound my wife made. He wasn't deaf, **just stubborn.** You had better believe things changed for him after that. He definitely started to listen to his mother; especially since he also said, "DADA," for the very first time during that experience.

During that time frame, a family friend, who'd been certified in infant CPR, started babysitting for our youngest son, allowing us some time together. This was incredibly scary for the first couple of nights; finally though we did get comfortable with it, after a while. The interesting thing that we learned was that she spoke Spanish to our youngest son and he responded appropriately to her. How do you like that! He'd ignore my wife when she spoke but eagerly responded to the sitter when she spoke to him in a different language. My wife was not very happy about that. She and our youngest son came to an understanding though soon after these experiences.

## 5 FOURTH MONTH

About now, we were starting to really get settled into a routine. The monitor was only going off, at night, once a week and the baby was pulling himself out of it. Thank God for that loud tone. True, our sleep was getting interrupted still, but he was bringing himself back on his own with the tone. It was worth it.

It was once again our turn to answer the hotline calls. After the first month, the other parents of the support group had volunteered to alternate answering the hotline calls and our turn had come up again.

One night we got a phone call from a hospital nurse on the opposite side of Phoenix. She told us that a resident had just informed a family that their child was a potential SIDS baby and they could do nothing about it, except let the baby die. Needless to say, my wife was a little unhappy about that statement. The first thing she did was ask if the doctor was available. The nurse went and got him, and I proceeded to hear her one-sided conversation. I couldn't believe it. Her first statement went something like this: "How dare you speak to those parents that way; to not give them some kind of hope! That's criminal!" She then told the doctor that she didn't care what he had to say, she wanted to speak to the parents. He obviously didn't know what to do, so he handed the phone off to the mother of the baby in question. It took my wife about two hours to convince the mother that there was hope for their child and not to give up trying. She did tell her that it was not going to be easy but every second of the child's life was worth it.

Another phone call came about 2:00 a.m. in the morning. It turned out that a child had just died of SIDS. The hospital where the child died had no idea how to deal with the mother's grief, so we got a call. To watch my wife during this phone call was amazing. When they started talking the mother was full of grief, questions and guilt.

She had no idea why it happened. She began listing the things that she could have done differently; which she felt may have kept her baby alive. To this day I cannot tell you what my wife said to her. All I know is that it was pure emotion. She completely bared herself to this woman, this mother, about losing a child. They both cried; heart-wrenching tears for their individual losses. Eventually, in some small way the mother began the processor understanding that there was nothing she could've done to prevent her child's death. They both relished the time they'd had with their children; my wife and this other mother. When the call was over my wife was completely drained. I had to help her to bed and beg her to try to get some sleep. I saw in that moment, that once again because of helping someone, she'd in turn helped herself a little bit more with dealing with her pain.

Our son was now four months old and we had to discuss getting him circumcised. The doctors had warned us that this needed to be done soon and we had nothing to worry about with his SIDS symptoms. For some reason we just didn't quite feel comfortable until now. So we scheduled it.

It turned out that the procedure was going to happen the same day that I was to receive a ten-year award from the place where I worked. My wife convinced me to go to the award banquet and tried to assure me that everything would be all right. So I reluctantly left. Assuring myself that she had the phone number of the hotel where the award ceremony was taking place.

Everything seemed to be going so well, for a while. About halfway into the ceremony I received a phone call. My wife was frantic. The monitor would not stop going off, and she'd tried to revive the baby twice. I put the phone down and left. I was shocked, terrified and frantic to get to them.

Now you have to remember, this hotel was thirty miles across town from where we lived. All I remember is getting into the car and arriving at the house. Don't ask me how fast I drove, or how I got there, I just did.

I ran into the house to find my wife sitting on our sofa with our son in her arms. She looked at me and said, "He is fine, I just wanted to hold him." The weight of the world just left my shoulders with that sight.

I then proceeded to ask her what happened. She told me how she'd revived him a couple of times, and how she'd almost lost him. But he came back. Thank God. I was floored, humbled but most of all overwhelmingly thankful at the outcome. It took us a couple of days to recover from that experience, but we did. Every day was becoming more important now.

One fine Saturday afternoon, our oldest son and I were watching TV while his mother was making something for supper. All of the sudden we heard two loud bangs upstairs in the baby's room. Needless to say, all three of us were up there within seconds. And there, with the side of the crib down, the mattress off at an angle, sat our youngest child, in one corner of the mattress. He had his hands out and in them were the screws from the crib. All he said was, "DADA." I couldn't believe it, my wife couldn't believe it.

She calmly turned to me and said, "You'd better figure out how to put those back in so he cannot do that again."

At that point I didn't know what to say, except, "This child is going to be interesting when he gets older."

## 6 FIFTH MONTH

At the start of this month, my wife had talked to her mother in Vermont a lot on the phone. It was bothering her that her mother might never get to know her youngest grandson. You have to understand that my mother-in-law does not fly. I don't know why, but she doesn't.

So my wife came up with a plan. She and the boys would go back to Vermont for a visit. The only problem was that I couldn't go with them because of previous work commitments. So, she suggested that they would go without me. My mind was instantly, selfishly I knew, filled with relief. No monitor for a couple of weeks, I might even get a full night of sleep.

When the day came for their trip, I found out how difficult it was going to be for me to sleep without them. Not knowing what was going on with the baby was driving me nuts and that was only in the first couple of hours. The doctor was okay with the baby taking the trip as long as my wife brought the monitor and she kept a close eye on him during the flight.

As soon as they got there, my wife called me. She was laughing hysterically. I asked her what happened but she continued laughing. It turns out that when she got off the plane in Montreal, her mother and her stepfather were waiting for them. The baby was being carried in a backpack on my wife's back. As soon as she could, her mother took the baby out of the backpack. He then proceeded to wrap both of his arms around her neck and plant his teeth into her nose. To this day, I still believe that he was trying, in his own way, to kiss her; that's my story and I am sticking to it. My mother-in-law proceeded to scream, "Get him off, get him off!"

Well it took my wife and her stepfather both to loosen the grip around her neck. And by the way, he was still smiling. At that point my mother-in-law said, "I could really dislike you if you weren't so darn cute."

Obviously, I was calling every day to get updates on how everyone was doing. You can forget the idea of a full night of sleep; it never happened as long as they were away.

The first day they were there, my wife called laughing again. My only question was, "What did he do this time?"

It turns out that my mother-in-law wanted to give my wife some extra time to sleep in. Her plan was to get the baby out of bed before his mother woke up and play with him.

Good plan, great intentions. But... she forgot about the monitor; in fact, she didn't even give it a thought, until it went off. My wife told me that after it started going off, that her mother could only yell, **"Ahhhhhh, what do I do? What do I do?"** Needless to say my mother-in-law never tried to surprise my wife again. In fact, to this day she still swears that alarm could wake the dead. And do you know what, I agree.

According to my wife, things calmed down for a couple of days after that incident. It was four days later when she told me about another incident that was very interesting. You have to understand that my mother-in-law was living in a trailer at the time. It was a three-bedroom trailer and they were small rooms with a very narrow hallway leading to the back bedroom, where my wife and the boys were sleeping. Everything was fine until one afternoon, while the baby was down for his nap, the alarm went off.

Both my wife and her mother started running for the alarm; my mother-in-law was in front, she was even calling out the baby's name like she was supposed to. About halfway down the hallway, she stopped dead in her tracks and said, "Oh my God, I don't know what to do when I get there." That didn't bother my wife at all. She proceeded to climb up her mother's back to get to the baby. My mother-in-law finally got her off and moved aside enough for my wife to get through. Would you believe our son was lying with the monitor lead in his hand and a big smile on his face? At that point, he now had one unhappy grandmother on his hands. She was still shaking from the realization that she wouldn't have known what to do if she was alone with him. She was very careful from that point on.

On the Saturday during that visit, my mother-in-law planned a family dinner so everyone could see my wife and the boys. Her brother, Randy, and her sister, Donna, both came with their families. They all sat at the table with my wife in the back corner surrounded by nieces and nephews. Our niece Chastity was sitting to her left. Well, the microwave alarm went off when it had completed cooking something. As luck would have it the microwave alarm sounded just like a monitor alarm. My wife went hysterical! She tried to climb over our niece any way she could. And all Chastity could do was stare at her with her mouth wide open. It was my wife's mother who finally calmed her down. She kept yelling, "Deb, it's the microwave! It's the microwave!"

Needless to say, my wife was very embarrassed when it sank in. Poor Chastity, it took my wife a good half hour of apologies before her niece would even consider talking to her.

I couldn't wait for them to get home. When they finally did it was great. Alarms and all, it was great to have them back.

## 7 SIXTH MONTH

Well, the monitor is not going off very often anymore and we are getting sleep for a change now. It seemed like we had passed the critical stage of this whole thing. Thank God.

Don't get me wrong, he still managed to set the alarms off when he wanted attention, but it was no longer because he would quit breathing in his sleep. Obviously, though, we weren't letting our guard down. That monitor was still the center of our life.

My wife was still giving talks to anyone interested in this illness. I was still going with her as support. A lot of these talks were becoming routine for me; so I would let my mind wander. During one of these sessions I realized something. What came to me was that my life up to this point really had no meaning.

You have to understand that I attended a Catholic

grammar school and high school. Prior to graduation from that facility we'd been asked to put down what we thought our life's goals were. Mine was that:  I wanted to have a street named after me, I wanted to be in the hall of fame, and I wanted to play professional sports. When the nun asked me what sport I was going to play though I couldn't answer her. Needless to say, my classmates had a good time razing me about my goals.

But looking back at it, at this time in my life, I realized that:  I had three streets named after me, I had been named to the Drum Corps Hall of Fame twice, and had played in four professional racquetball tournaments.  Besides that, professionally I was considered a leading technical person in a company of 120 thousand. But…you know what? None of that mattered anymore. The only thing that mattered to me was my family. Wow, I had finally gotten it. Without them I was nothing and with them I was everything.

It was during this time that the support organization got setup with name and structure. The name we came up with was P.O.C.O.M. It stood for Parents of Children on Monitors.

One couple, Charlie and Julie, had volunteered to head fund-raising. Another couple, Mike and Stacy, chose to lead the disbursement of funds.  My wife and I ended up with organizing talks and communications.

Almost immediately, we became very successful at raising funds. The disbursement of these funds ended up being 100% used for the support of monitoring equipment and medications for our 170 member families in Arizona. Because of these facts, we thought we needed to become associated with a national organization to enhance our support activities. Boy, did we get an education. It turns out that all the associated national organizations only wanted to talk to us if we would turn the control of our funds over to them. We couldn't do that!

It was about now that we were approached by a unique individual. He was the facilitator of an organization call the Patrick Murphy Foundation. It turns out that this organization gave financial aid to families of terminally ill children that the other national organizations wouldn't support. He was excited to have us join his organization, even with the fact that our children had a great chance of survival. With this organization we were able to contribute to the building of the Ronald McDonald House in Phoenix with the help of the McDonald's corporation.

At this same time in our life, the baby was getting heavier now. In fact, it was difficult to carry him in your arms because of the weight he'd gained. So, I started carrying him on my shoulders. This worked. It displaced the weight and it kept him happy. This worked until the day we walked into a toy store. As I passed some very colorful toys, I found out why you do not want to do this. Once he noticed those brightly colored toys, he grabbed my hair with both hands and tried to steer me back to the toys that had caught his eye. Nothing but pain! My wife was no help; she just laughed and suggested that I give in and go where he wanted me to.

Any experienced parent will tell you that once the child determines where you are going in a toy store you're in trouble. I learned that the hard way that day. He was into everything and it took me forever to straighten up the displays. So, I learned a very important lesson that day. No more shoulders in stores.

## 8 SEVENTH MONTH

One of the activities we tried to keep consistent was having monthly meetings with the parents of other children on monitors. These meetings took place in someone's home and the location was different month to month. It was our turn to host the discussion with as many local parents as we could get to come.

For this meeting, we had a visitor from the company that provided the monitors coming to speak with us. This guest brought about twenty couples to our home. You have to remember, we had a very small townhouse and forty people in the downstairs living room was very crowded.

At these events, the men usually migrated to the kitchen while the wives stayed in the living room area. When the representative from the monitor company showed up, he was seated in the middle of the living room with our wives. Everything went real well for the majority of the meeting until the representative of Monitor Company said, "You mothers have to stop your babies from teething on the leads and pads for the monitor." Right after that statement came out of his mouth all the fathers just looked at each other and calmly told him that he was on his own.

Our wives didn't stop going after him for a full ten minutes. And guess who was leading the barrage. Yes, my wife. She kept asking him, "Do you have children? Do you? Have you ever been able to stop them from teething?" After the wives got through with him, he was handing all of them extra pads, and leads off of his truck. He even then and there promised to visit each household to make sure that the units were working properly. The husbands almost felt sorry for him. I said *almost*. It was ugly.

It was also during these meetings that we discussed the stress level that we all lived with. The doctors were constantly reminding us that the divorce rate among couples with children on monitors was currently between 75 and 80%. We all shared different ways that we dealt with the stress. Now according to my wife, I didn't deal with it. And she proceeded to tell all the couples of perhaps the biggest mistake I've ever made in our marriage.

We've definitely had our arguments throughout the course or our son's illness and I was losing a lot of them. She would say that she was trying to get me to grow up. She was probably right even if at the time I didn't agree—boy, did I try to fight that. (Without success, I might add.)

During one of these **discussions,** I decided to respond to her the same way my father had responded to my mother when she was angry with him. So, I calmly looked at her and said, "When you decide to discuss this calmly and rationally, let me know." Right after it came out of my mouth I remembered how my mother reacted. Immediately, I realized that this was a big mistake. Boy, did I hear about that one.

Don't get me wrong, our relationship was not always easy. I remember a lot of days walking in from work, meeting my wife on her way out saying, "He's your son, take care of him!" This did not go over very well with me at first but I understood. She would window shop for about an hour and then revived from some alone time, come home to be with us. Of course I always got the usual questions: "Did you feed the boys? Did you clean up? Did you change the baby's diaper?" That last one was the toughest for me to get consistently right. But I learned.

We all deal with stress differently. My wife and I were lucky, we were able to explain our feelings to each other and let them out. That is of course after a couple of months of her trying to teach me how. Male ego. Don't get me wrong, it wasn't pretty, but we always ended up understanding what it was. Stress.

The other fathers were all different on how they dealt with their stress. One even came up with something that could be a benefit for the children. He'd designed a bed that would not allow an infant to get into REM sleep (Rapid Eye Movement, the time when most of these infants would stop breathing). It would vibrate and bring the baby out of REM. The concept was good. The problem was that each child reached REM at different times. So we designed a variable timer to be set to each child.

It was these kinds of activities that kept us all going in our support group. The daily activities were something that we were all trying to enhance.

# 9 EIGHTH MONTH

The baby was getting older now, he was starting to crawl and investigate everything. This is typically when a good father decides to baby-proof their home. I considered myself a good father but I wasn't going to do it until absolutely I had to. My wife just laughed at me and said, "You have got another thing coming if you think that's going to work." Of course, being a male I didn't believe her.

Boy was I going to be shown just how wrong I was! It all started the day he crawled into the kitchen and opened the cabinet where she kept the pans. I don't know about you but the sound of a baby banging pan covers on the floor gets to me after a while. So I brought him back into the living room and put him down to play with him. Well, that didn't last long and he was right back into the pan covers. This time I closed the cabinet and wouldn't let him get into it. This almost worked until he noticed my wife's corner hutch, where she had her expensive milk glass pieces. Once I realized what he was after, the rest of the day he spent with me holding him. You can bet that went over real well with him.

As soon as I could, I went and bought some baby locks to put on the cabinets and my wife's hutch; along with a gate to the stairs going to the bedrooms. To this day, I remember putting those locks on with a screwdriver as tight as I possibly could. I didn't want another crib incident. When the baby got up from his nap, he started to investigate the locks. First, he looked at them, and then twisted his head from side to side, looking them over from all angles. I figured everything was safe. So, I relaxed in the living room. The next thing I heard was a loud *snap!* I went running into the kitchen. There in front of the corner hutch was my youngest son with the remnants of a baby lock in his hand. He'd torn it right out. It took a while for me to get everything out of the hutch and the cabinet for the pans, but I did it. It took even longer for me to admit to my wife that she was right. But I did that too.

Our youngest son amazed the doctors, especially the lead doctor on his case. It turns out that this particular doctor was a leading researcher in SIDS and was writing a book about his findings. He ended up asking for our permission to write a chapter about our youngest son. We agreed.

Whenever the doctor would see him, he always

had the same comment about him. He'd say that he loved our child because no matter what you did to him, he just keeps smiling. It also surprised the doctor that the baby didn't take much from anyone. According to the doctor, if you did something to the baby that he didn't like, he'd find a way to get even. I can believe it. I wonder where he got that from.

Part of our function in the support group was to attend functions designed to raise money. One of these functions was being put on by the Blue Knights of the Phoenix Police Department, don't feel bad I didn't know who they were either until it was explained to me. I found out, much to my surprise, that they're members of a motorcycle unit in the Phoenix Police Department. They get pledges to ride their motorcycles in order to give the money that they receive from it to specific groups. Today was our turn.

All during the day, they stopped by to talk to us. The idea was for them to understand what our organization was all about. It seems like every one of the riders couldn't get over our youngest son's attitude and constant smile. At the end of the day, they let us know that for the rest of the year our son was the poster child for this illness that they would be riding for.

## 10 NINTH MONTH

During this time, my wife and I had finally finished a pamphlet that we'd been working on to help the other families with children on monitors. When we showed the document to the doctors and the nurses we were surprised by their reaction to it.

First of all, they wanted to help by inserting the correct medical jargon and explanations. The also recommended that we send the pamphlet to a specific corporation to get it published. We didn't think the document was that good, but it was needed to help families in this situation.

We took their suggestions and did get a response from that corporation. It surprised us. They wanted to publish our document entitled Living with Infant Apnea. The only thing they asked was that we sign over the rights to the document since we didn't want to earn any profits from it. We agreed. Soon after, we were pleasantly surprised to find out that this document was translated into seven different languages and released all over the world. What a feeling that was, to know that people all over the world could be helped with a small document that we had created.

About this time, we were getting fantastic reports from the doctors. They'd been telling us that it appeared that our youngest son was no longer considered a threat for SIDS. Obviously, we weren't completely ready to accept this diagnosis. So, we continued to use the monitor when he was placed into his crib.

Within a week of the message from the doctors, the monitor company started calling us to ask when they could come and get the equipment. You can just imagine our reaction. N**ever!** We fought over this issue a lot during those days. One day my wife was ready to give it up and the next she wasn't. I was the same way. Through all of this, our oldest son didn't want the monitor to go either. As far as he was concerned it was keeping his little brother alive and it should never leave.

After about two weeks of this, my wife called the monitor company and told them that she was putting the equipment outside and they had an hour to come and get it. Guess What? They came and got it. I couldn't believe she really done this. After all that piece of equipment had become so important to our youngest son's existence.

Now I was back to standing next to his crib at night until I was satisfied that he was breathing correctly. Fortunately, that didn't last long. My wife finally convinced me to trust him, so I did.

## 11 THIRTY-TWO YEARS LATER

It's been quite awhile since the incident of our discovery of our son's illness and the months culminating the battle to overcome it. You're probably wondering why I waited so long to write about this. The reason is simple, every time I'd think about writing this book I'd remember the emotions that came along with this experience. Even today, I still feel a lot of anxiety talking about this subject. The first chapter of this document was written in January 1982 when it happened. After that, I wasn't able to revisit those emotions again until now.

After all of this time, I thought it would finally be appropriate to see where the incidents of SIDS were compared to the 1980's. Remember, in the 1980's it was estimated that 7000 infants died of SIDS each year around the world with 2500 being accounted for in the US. I was looking forward to that number decreasing with time and research.

The following information was found on the CDC (Center for Disease Control) in the US. It is estimated that in 2012 that 4000 infants died of what could be attributed to SIDS. I continued reading. It turns out that many more children die of SIDS in a year than all who die of cancer, heart disease, pneumonia, child abuse, AIDS, cystic fibrosis, and muscular dystrophy combined.

SIDS is responsible for more deaths than any other cause in childhood for babies one month to one year of age, claiming 150,000 victims in the United States in this generation alone.

While there are still no adequate medical explanations for SIDS deaths, current theories include: (1) stress in a normal baby, caused by infections or other factors; (2) a birth defect; (3) failure to develop; and/or (4) a critical period when all babies are especially vulnerable, such as a time of rapid growth.

These are some of the facts that I thought would be important to someone reading about SIDS for the first time.

What SIDS is not:

SIDS is not caused by external suffocation.

SIDS is not contagious

SIDS does not cause pain or suffering in the infant

SIDS is not new, it is referenced in the Old Testament.

There was another section on the site which mentioned that only 2250 cases of SIDS were recorded last year in the US. Now, that was a very encouraging piece of information. It's about time that the deaths were reduced. It's obvious that they (the medical profession) still have no idea of the cause, or any potential cure. It's clear that they're working on it. I salute them for that.

Our experience was one of prevention. And yet I am still very thankful for it. If you speak to anyone in the medical profession, they would tell you that our son was not a SIDS child because he lived. In fact, they're right. He was what they call a near-miss SIDS child, all the symptoms without the outcome.

They say it takes a village to bring up a family. Well, we had ours and I am very thankful for it.

One of most impressive things that happened to use while we were in Arizona was the fact that out of the 170 families with children on monitors, we did **not** lose one single child while we were there.

We're now living in Vermont and enjoying every minute of it. I still say that same prayer every night that I started during our first month on the monitor. Only now, it includes the grandchildren. And I no longer say it until I fall asleep.

We had returned to Vermont in order for me to fulfill a promise I made to my wife thirty-three years ago. Namely, that I would bring her back to her home someday to live; I kept that promise and it feels good.

Across the living room from me is my wife, watching television while I am working on the computer. She's still that same beautiful woman I married. I, on the other hand, have aged tremendously and I claim that she and the boys did it to me. That's my story and I am sticking to it.

To this day, I still can't believe that we lived through that experience. It was the scariest thing I had ever been part of as well as the greatest thing I had ever been part of. We both grew through it; but without her I would not have survived it.

Our oldest son now lives in Vermont and has children of his own. His youngest just turned eight-years-old and he is a proud father.

The screen saver on our computer is a picture of myself, our youngest son, and his seven-year old son who has a devilish twinkle in his eyes. His son's name is Kaeleb.

# ABOUT THE AUTHOR

The author was born and raised in Westfield, Massachusetts. He is the second of four brothers. While growing up in the 50's and the 60's, he experienced events that he held deep inside him until years later. When the time was right, he started writing about them.

He spent time in the military from 1968 to 1971. That experience left a lasting impression on him. When he left the military, he started working in the computer field. Both he and his wife have lived it multiple locations throughout the country because of that experience.

When he retired, he realized that he had a need to express himself and began writing. Currently, the author and his wife reside in the "smallest city" in Vermont due to a promise he made to her prior to their marriage thirty-three years ago.

# MORE BOOKS BY MICHAEL WALSH

Wizards of Now
Just Some Old Man
Largo
The Whetstone Chronicle
Eddie's Method
Gillbrath
James of Elan
Key of Wands
Knights of Forever
Tyme of Now

Made in the USA
Lexington, KY
26 July 2014